GREEK
COOKBOOK

Authentic Food from Greece in 75 Easy Recipes.

Contents

Introduction

Greek food has a long history and is known for its wide scope of dishes, from delicate barbecued meats and fiery plates of mixed greens. As the southernmost country in Europe, terrain Greece and the islands around it encounter a Mediterranean environment ideal for viticulture. Also, its current position in the Aegean has given direct access to fresh seafood for the previous 10,000 years.

The Greek eating regimen has changed from the beginning of time. It depends on wheat, wine, and olive oil. Since Greece is near Constantinople (Istanbul), it profited from the reality that it was at the center of worldwide exchange. Bunches of new spices and flavors came to Greece. Just as this, Greece got some new vegetables to explore different avenues of its cuisine. This was a period of worldwide exchange, with Constantinople in the middle, which clarifies why Greek and Turkish food are so comparable. It is most likely not unexpected to discover that advanced Greek food has its foundations from old Greece. Fish is ordinarily eaten more than meat, as it is more generally accessible. Consider how Greece has such a lot of water around it. This added to the wellbeing variable of the eating routine, as fish contains significant enhancements like omega 3.

Conventional Greek food is described by top-notch fixings that are added to it. Greek gastronomy is one of the best of the world's exemplary cooking styles. It is usually called a foodie's paradise. The main ingredients of Greek cooking incorporate olive oil, shrimp, spices (thyme, rosemary, and oregano are the most well-known), cheddar, tomatoes, ham, sheep, pork, fish, and wine. All the ingredients used in Greek food can be easily found at any exotic or general store.

Each city, town, and island in Greece has its own culinary fortes. Provincial dishes are an ideal approach to taste the cuisine. Santorini, specifically, fuses extraordinary items like fava beans, cherry tomatoes, and the assyrtiko grapes into its gastronomy. Greeks love meat, yet they additionally comprehend the worth of an even feast. No customary Greek feast is complete without a huge and fiery serving of mixed greens.

During the 1900s, Greeks lived longer and had lower paces of constant infection than the remainder of the world. This is reasonable because of their eating routine, brimming with fish, organic products, vegetables, beans, grains and solid fats. The Mediterranean eating routine depends on the customary Greek eating regimen and other comparable food cuisines of nations. Examination recommends that the Mediterranean Diet can diminish your danger of respiratory failure, stroke, diabetes, heftiness, and sudden death.

Hummus is a well-known plunge or spread all through the Mediterranean and the Middle East. Exploration recommends that eating hummus may assist with weight reduction, glucose control, and heart wellbeing. This is halfway because of its primary ingredient, i.e., chickpeas, which are otherwise called garbanzo beans. They are a fantastic wellspring of protein and fiber. Dolmades are full of grape leaves filled in as a starter or as a main dish. They are ordinarily loaded down with rice, spices, and at times the meat. The stuffing can shift, modifying their fat and calorie substance. Red grape leaves may further develop blood dissemination in individuals with ongoing blood deficiency, a condition wherein blood struggles flowing through the blood vessels. So, in short, all the ingredients used in Greek cuisine are extremely delicious and healthy at the same time. You can opt for this Greek lifestyle to stay healthy and fit for life.

You will learn various different recipes originated from Greece in this book. This book contains 75 recipes that are traditionally cooked in Greece. The recipe section will include breakfast, lunch, dinner, snacks, vegetarian and sweet dishes. All these recipes are detailed with easy-to-follow instructions and detailed ingredients that help you out in cooking by yourself at home. So, start reading this amazing book now!

Chapter 1: The Famous Greek Breakfast Recipes

Breakfast in Greece has a novel history. Following are traditional breakfast recipes that Greek people around the world love:

1.1 Greek Omelet Casserole Recipe

Preparation Time: 30 minutes
Cooking Time: 30 minutes
Serving: 4

Ingredients:

- Twelve large eggs
- Twelve ounces of artichoke salad
- Eight ounces of freshly cut spinach
- One tablespoon of fresh dill
- Four teaspoons of olive oil
- One teaspoon of dried oregano
- Two cloves of chopped garlic
- Two cups of whole milk
- Five ounces of sun-dried tomatoes
- One cup of crumbled feta cheese
- One teaspoon of lemon pepper
- One teaspoon of salt
- One teaspoon of pepper

Instructions:
1. Take a large bowl.
2. Add the eggs into the bowl.
3. Beat the eggs for about five minutes.
4. Take another bowl and add the pepper, lemon pepper, fresh dill, dried oregano, and salt into the bowl.
5. Mix all the ingredients well.

6. Add the olive oil and spinach into the egg bowl.
7. Mix the ingredients well and add the chopped garlic and the rest of the ingredients.
8. Mix all the ingredients of both the bowls together.
9. Add the mixture to a greased baking dish.
10. Bake the casserole for twenty-five to thirty minutes.
11. Dish out the casserole when done.
12. The dish is ready to be served.

1.2 Greek Cheese Pie with Nuts and Honey Recipe

Preparation Time: 20 minutes
Cooking Time: 40 minutes
Serving: 4

Ingredients:

- Eight ounces of feta cheese
- One pack of phyllo sheets
- One teaspoon of dried mint
- Half cup of chopped nuts (of your choice)
- One cup of honey thyme
- One cup of strained Greek yoghurt
- Seven ounces of butter

Instructions:
1. Take a large bowl.
2. Add the butter into it and beat well.
3. Add the Greek yoghurt and feta cheese into the butter bowl.
4. Mix the ingredients well.
5. Add the dried mint into the bowl and mix well.
6. Spread the phyllo sheets in a greased baking tray.
7. Add the cheese mixture into the phyllo sheets and cover it with more phyllo sheets.
8. Bake the pie for about forty minutes.
9. Dish out the pie.
10. Drizzle the honey thyme on top of the pie.

11. Garnish the dish with chopped nuts
12. The dish is ready to be served.

1.3 Greek Avocado Toast Recipe

Preparation Time: 30 minutes
Cooking Time: 20 minutes
Serving: 4

Ingredients:

- Half cup of lemon juice
- Four slices of bread
- Half cup of cherry tomatoes
- Half cup of extra-virgin olive oil
- Half cup of crumbled cheese
- Crushed red chilies
- Half cup of chopped cucumber
- A quarter cup of dill
- Half cup of Kalamata olives
- Two cups of chopped avocado
- A pinch of salt
- A pinch of black pepper

Instructions:

1. Take a large bowl.
2. Add all the ingredients except the bread slices.
3. Mix all the ingredients.
4. Toast the bread slices
5. Spread the mixture on top of the bread slices.
6. Your dish is ready to be served.

1.4 Greek Scrambled Eggs Recipe

Preparation Time: 10 minutes
Cooking Time: 15 minutes
Serving: 2

Ingredients:

- Two tablespoons of olive oil
- Two large eggs
- One ripe cherry tomato
- A pinch of salt
- A pinch of black pepper

Instructions:
1. Take a large pan.
2. Add the olive oil into the pan.
3. Add the tomatoes and salt into the pan.
4. Cook the tomatoes well, and then add the black pepper into the pan.
5. Break the eggs into the pan.
6. Scramble the ingredients well.
7. Dish out when the eggs are done
8. Your dish is ready to be served.

1.5 Greek Fried Eggs with Potato and Feta Recipe

Preparation Time: 10 minutes
Cooking Time: 15 minutes
Serving: 2

Ingredients:

- Two tablespoons of olive oil
- Two large eggs
- One chopped potato
- Sixty grams of feta cheese
- A pinch of salt
- A pinch of black pepper

Instructions:
1. Take a large pan.
2. Add the olive oil into the pan.
3. Add the potatoes and salt into the pan.
4. Cook the potatoes well and then add the black pepper into the pan.
5. Break the eggs into the pan.

6. Add the crumbled feta cheese on top.
7. Cook the ingredients well on both sides.
8. Dish out when the eggs are done
9. Your dish is ready to be served.

1.6 Greek Sesame Bread Rings Recipe

Preparation Time: 20 minutes
Cooking Time: 40 minutes
Serving: 4

Ingredients:

- Two cups of flour
- Three tablespoons of olive oil
- Two teaspoons of salt
- Half teaspoon of yeast
- One teaspoon of sugar
- One cup of sesame seeds
- One cup of lukewarm water

Instructions:
1. Take a large bowl.
2. Add the sugar, yeast, and lukewarm water into the bowl.
3. Mix well and keep aside until bubbles are formed.
4. Add the flour and salt into the mixture.
5. Knead the dough well and start forming ring structures from the dough mixture.
6. Add the sesame seeds on top of the rings and place the rings on a baking tray.
7. Bake the dish for about thirty minutes.
8. Your dish is ready to be served.

1.7 Greek Breakfast Ladenia (Flatbread with Tomatoes) Recipe

Preparation Time: 30 minutes
Cooking Time: 10 minutes
Serving: 4

Ingredients:

- Two cups of flour

- Three tablespoons of olive oil
- Two teaspoons of salt
- Half teaspoon of yeast
- One teaspoon of sugar
- One cup of cherry tomatoes
- Two teaspoons of dried oregano
- One cup of sliced onions
- One cup of lukewarm water

Instructions:
1. Take a large bowl.
2. Add the sugar, yeast, and lukewarm water into the bowl.
3. Mix well and keep aside until bubbles are formed.
4. Add the flour and salt into the mixture.
5. Knead the dough well and start forming round flatbread from the dough mixture.
6. Add the sliced onion and cherry tomatoes on top of the bread and place the bread dough on a baking tray.
7. Bake the dish for about thirty minutes.
8. Your dish is ready to be served.

1.8 Greek Breakfast Rice Pudding (Rizogalo) Recipe

Preparation Time: 20 minutes
Cooking Time: 30 minutes
Serving: 4

Ingredients:

- Two cups of whole milk
- Two cups of water
- Four tablespoons of cornstarch
- Four tablespoons of white sugar
- Half cup of rice
- A quarter teaspoon of cinnamon powder

Instructions:

1. Take a large saucepan.
2. Add the water and whole milk.
3. Let the liquid boil for five minutes.
4. Add the rice and sugar into the milk mixture.
5. Cook all the ingredients well for thirty minutes or until it starts to get thick.
6. Add the cinnamon powder on top.
7. The dish is ready to be served.

1.9 Greek Breakfast Egg Muffins Recipe

Preparation Time: 20 minutes
Cooking Time: 20 minutes
Serving: 4

Ingredients:

- Half cup of sun-dried tomatoes
- Ten eggs
- A quarter cup of olives
- One cup of crumbled cheese
- A quarter cup of cream

Instructions:

1. Take a large bowl.
2. Add all the ingredients into the bowl.
3. Mix everything well.
4. Pour the egg mixture into a greased muffin tray.
5. Bake the muffins for twenty to thirty minutes.
6. Dish out the muffins.
7. The dish is ready to be served.

1.10 Greek Breakfast Egg Skillet with Vegetables and Feta Recipe

Preparation Time: 10 minutes
Cooking Time: 15 minutes
Serving: 2

Ingredients:

- Two tablespoons of olive oil
- Two large eggs
- One ripe cherry tomato
- Two cups of chopped baby spinach

- One cup of chopped onion
- One cup of bell pepper
- A quarter cup of crumbled feta cheese
- A pinch of salt
- A pinch of black pepper

Instructions:
1. Take a large pan.
2. Add the olive oil into the pan.
3. Add the onion and salt into the pan.
4. Cook the onions well, and then add the black pepper into the pan.
5. Add the baby spinach and bell pepper into the mixture.
6. Cook the ingredients well for about five minutes.
7. Break the eggs into the pan.
8. Cook the ingredients well.
9. Dish out when the eggs are done.
10. Garnish the dish with crumbled feta cheese.
11. Your dish is ready to be served.

1.11 Greek Breakfast Pitas Recipe

Preparation Time: 10 minutes
Cooking Time: 15 minutes
Serving: 2

Ingredients:

- Two tablespoons of olive oil
- Two slices of pita bread
- Two large eggs
- One ripe cherry tomato
- Two cups of chopped baby spinach
- One cup of chopped onion
- Half cup of chopped basil
- One cup of bell pepper
- A quarter cup of crumbled feta cheese
- A pinch of salt

- A pinch of black pepper
- A bunch of chopped cilantro

Instructions:
1. Take a large pan.
2. Add the olive oil into the pan.
3. Add the onion and salt into the pan.
4. Cook the onions well, and then add the black pepper into the pan.
5. Add the baby spinach and bell pepper into the mixture.
6. Cook the ingredients well for about five minutes.
7. Break the eggs into the pan.
8. Cook the ingredients well.
9. Dish out when the eggs are done.
10. Let the eggs cool down, and then add the crumbled feta cheese into it.
11. Mix well.
12. Heat the pita bread.
13. Cut a hole into the bread and add the cooked mixture into it.
14. Garnish the bread with chopped cilantro.
15. Your dish is ready to be served.

Chapter 2: The Famous Greek Lunch Recipes

Classic Greek lunch recipes are extremely delicious and worth eating. Following are some classic Greek recipes that are rich in healthy nutrients, and you can easily make them with the detailed instructions list in each recipe:

2.1 Greek Classic Lemon Potatoes Recipe

Preparation Time: 30 minutes
Cooking Time: 25 minutes
Serving: 4

Ingredients:

- One cup of onion
- One cup of vegetable broth
- Half teaspoon of smoked paprika
- Two tablespoons of Dijon mustard
- Two teaspoons of white sugar
- Two tablespoons of olive oil
- Two cups of tomato paste
- One tablespoon of dried rosemary
- A pinch of salt
- A pinch of black pepper
- One teaspoon of dried thyme
- One pound of cauliflower florets
- Two tablespoons of minced garlic
- Half cup of dry white wine
- Half cup of lemon juice
- Half cup of cilantro

Instructions:
1. Take a large pan.
2. Add the olive oil and onion slices into it.
3. Fry the onion slices and then dish it out.
4. Add the garlic, potato pieces, lemon juice, and spices into the pan.

5. Cook the potato pieces in the spices for five to ten minutes.
6. Add the rest of the ingredients into the mixture.
7. Cook the mixture until it starts boiling.
8. Bring the heat to low and cover the pan with a lid.
9. After ten minutes, remove the lid.
10. Check the potatoes before dishing them out.
11. Crumble the cooked onion slices on top before serving.
12. Your dish is ready to be served.

2.2 Greek Salad Recipes

Preparation Time: 20 minutes
Cooking Time: 15 minutes
Serving: 2

Ingredients:

For the dressing:
- Half teaspoon of kosher salt
- Two teaspoons of freshly ground black pepper
- A quarter cup of red wine vinegar
- Half cup of olive oil
- Two tablespoons of minced garlic
- Two teaspoons of fresh oregano
- Half teaspoon of dried oregano

For salad:
- One cup of feta cheese
- Half cup of parmesan cheese
- Half pound of bread slices
- Half teaspoon of minced garlic
- Two tablespoons of olive oil
- Half cup of Kalamata olives
- One cup of red-orange bell pepper
- One cup of English cucumber
- One cup of cherry tomatoes

Instructions:
1. Take a small bowl.
2. Add the olive oil and minced garlic into it.
3. Mix it well and spread it on the bread slices.
4. Add the parmesan cheese on top of the slices.

5. Bake the slices for ten minutes.
6. Dish out the bread slices when they are done.
7. Take a large bowl.
8. Add the English cucumber, Kalamata olives, red-orange bell pepper, cherry tomatoes, and feta cheese into the bowl.
9. Mix everything well and set it aside.
10. Take a small bowl.
11. Add the olive oil, red wine vinegar, kosher salt, minced garlic, freshly crushed black pepper, fresh oregano, and dried oregano.
12. Mix everything well.
13. Pour this dressing on the prepared salad.
14. Mix everything well and add the toasted bread slices to the side.
15. Your dish is ready to be served.

2.3 Greek Chicken Gyros Recipe

Preparation Time: 10 minutes
Cooking Time: 30 minutes
Serving: 4

Ingredients:

- Four flatbreads
- Half cup of vegetable broth
- A quarter cup of lemon juice
- One cup of tzatziki sauce
- Half cup of sliced red onion
- Half cup of sliced tomatoes
- Half cup of romaine lettuce
- One tablespoon of minced garlic
- One cup of tomato paste
- Two tablespoons of olive oil
- One tablespoon of garlic powder
- One tablespoon of dried thyme
- Half teaspoon of ground cinnamon
- Two tablespoons of chili powder
- A quarter teaspoon of fresh nutmeg
- A pinch of sea salt

- Two cups of chicken pieces

Instructions:
1. Take a large pan.
2. Add the olive oil and garlic into the pan.
3. Add the oregano, tomato paste, smoked paprika, nutmeg, chili powder, thyme, and salt.
4. Add the vegetable broth, lemon juice, and chicken pieces into the pan.
5. Cook the ingredients well for about fifteen minutes.
6. Bake the flatbreads for about two to three minutes.
7. Cut the flatbreads in between to form a pouch structure.
8. Add the cooked mixture into the flatbread and line it with tzatziki sauce, romaine lettuce, sliced tomatoes, and red onions.
9. Your dish is ready to be served.

2.4 Greek Meatballs Recipe

Preparation Time: 10 minutes
Cooking Time: 20 minutes
Serving: 2

Ingredients:

- One chopped red onion
- Two minced garlic cloves
- A pinch of salt
- A pinch of black pepper
- Half cup of mint leaves
- Two cups of beef mince
- Half teaspoon of oregano
- One egg
- Two tablespoons of olive oil
- One cup of Greek yoghurt

Instructions:
1. Take a large bowl.
2. Add the beef mince, spices, mint, onion, garlic, and egg into the bowl.
3. Mix all the ingredients well and form round ball structures.
4. Fry the meatballs in olive oil until they turn golden brown.
5. Dish out the meatballs.
6. Serve the meatballs with Greek yoghurt on the side.
7. Your dish is ready to be served.

2.5 Greek Stuffed Peppers Recipe

Preparation Time: 10 minutes
Cooking Time: 20 minutes
Serving: 2

Ingredients:

- Half cup of cooked rice
- One cup of tomato paste
- Two tablespoons of unsalted butter
- Three tablespoons of granulated sugar
- Half cup of chopped carrots
- One teaspoon of minced ginger
- Two cups of mixed cheese
- Chopped fresh parsley
- Two tablespoons of olive oil
- One pound of green bell peppers
- Two cups of tomatoes
- A pinch of salt
- A pinch of black pepper
- Two cups of chopped potatoes
- One cup of chopped red onions
- One tablespoon of minced garlic
- Half cup of chopped zucchini

Instructions:
1. Take a large pan.
2. Add the butter and chopped onions into the pan.
3. Cook the onion until it turns soft.
4. Add the garlic and ginger as well as the chopped zucchini, chopped potatoes, tomatoes, tomato paste, and chopped carrots.
5. Cook the vegetables well for about ten minutes.
6. Add the granulated sugar, cooked rice, salt, and pepper.
7. Mix everything well and dish out.
8. Clean the bell peppers from inside and add the cooked mixture into it.
9. Add the mixed cheese on top and place the bell peppers on a greased baking tray.

10. Bake the bell peppers until the cheese turns light golden brown.
11. Garnish the bell peppers with freshly chopped parsley leaves.
12. Your dish is ready to be served.

2.6 Greek Bean Soup Recipe

Preparation Time: 30 minutes
Cooking Time: 30 minutes
Serving: 4

Ingredients:

- Half cup of chopped fresh thyme
- Half cup of chopped fresh oregano
- Half cup of chopped fresh chives
- One teaspoon of mixed spice powder
- Half teaspoon of smoked paprika
- One bay leaf
- A pinch of salt
- A pinch of black pepper
- Two tablespoons of olive oil
- One pound of beans
- Half tablespoon of chopped garlic
- Two cups of chopped tomatoes
- One cup of chopped onions
- One cup of chopped parsley
- One cup of vegetable stock
- One cup of water

Instructions:

1. Take a large pan.
2. Add the chopped onions and olive oil into it.
3. Mix the ingredients well.
4. Add the chopped garlic into the pan.
5. Add the tomatoes, oregano, bay leaf, salt, black pepper, thyme, smoked paprika, mix spice powder, and chives into the pan.
6. Cook the ingredients well.
7. Add the beans into the mixture.
8. Add the vegetable stock and water into the pan.
9. Mix the soup well.
10. Place a lid on top of the pan.
11. Cook the soup for ten to fifteen minutes.
12. Dish out the soup when the beans are done.

13.   Garnish the dish with chopped parsley on top.
14.   Your dish is ready to be served.

2.7 Greek Roasted Green Beans Recipe

Preparation Time: 30 minutes
Cooking Time: 20 minutes
Serving: 4

Ingredients:

- A pinch of salt
- A pinch of black pepper
- Four cups of diced green beans
- One cup of chopped onion
- Half tablespoon of chopped garlic,
- Three tablespoons of olive oil
- Two tablespoons of granulated sugar
- Two tablespoons of chopped parsley
- One tablespoon of smoked paprika
- Two tablespoons of fresh oregano
- Two tablespoons of fresh thyme
- Half cup of vegetable stock
- One cup of chopped tomatoes

Instructions:

1. Take a large pan.
2. Add the chopped onions and olive oil to it.
3. Mix the ingredients well.
4. Add the chopped garlic into the pan.
5. Add the tomatoes, oregano, salt, black pepper, granulated sugar, thyme, and smoked paprika into the pan.
6. Cook the ingredients well.
7. Add the diced green beans to the mixture.
8. Add the vegetable stock into the pan.
9. Mix the ingredients well.
10. Place a lid on top of the pan.
11. Cook the green beans for ten to fifteen minutes.
12. Dish out the food when the green beans are done.
13. Garnish the dish with chopped parsley on top.
14. Your dish is ready to be served.

2.8 Greek Lentil Soup Recipe

Preparation Time: 30 minutes
Cooking Time: 30 minutes
Serving: 4

Ingredients:

- A pinch of salt
- A pinch of black pepper
- Two tablespoons of olive oil
- One pound of mixed lentils
- Half tablespoon of chopped garlic
- Two cups of chopped tomatoes
- Half cup of chopped fresh thyme
- Half cup of chopped fresh oregano
- Half cup of chopped fresh chives
- One teaspoon of mixed spice powder
- Half teaspoon of smoked paprika
- One bay leaf
- One cup of chopped onions
- One cup of chopped parsley
- One cup of vegetable stock
- One cup of water

Instructions:
1. Take a large pan.
2. Add the chopped onions and olive oil into it.
3. Mix the ingredients well.
4. Add the chopped garlic into the pan.
5. Add the tomatoes, oregano, bay leaf, salt, black pepper, thyme, smoked paprika, mix spice powder, and chives into the pan.
6. Cook the ingredients well.
7. Add the lentils into the mixture.
8. Add the vegetable stock and water into the pan.
9. Mix the soup well.
10. Place a lid on top of the pan.
11. Cook the soup for ten to fifteen minutes.
12. Dish out the soup when the lentils are done.

13. Garnish the dish with chopped parsley on top.
14. Your dish is ready to be served.

2.9 Greek Chickpea Soup Recipe

Preparation Time: 30 minutes
Cooking Time: 30 minutes
Serving: 4

Ingredients:

- One cup of chopped onions
- One cup of chopped parsley
- One cup of vegetable stock
- One cup of water
- A pinch of salt
- A pinch of black pepper
- Two tablespoons of olive oil
- One pound of chickpeas
- Half tablespoon of chopped garlic
- Two cups of chopped tomatoes
- Half cup of chopped fresh thyme
- Half cup of chopped fresh oregano
- Half cup of chopped fresh chives
- One teaspoon of mixed spice powder
- Half teaspoon of smoked paprika
- One bay leaf

Instructions:
1. Take a large pan.
2. Add the chopped onions and olive oil into it.
3. Mix the ingredients well.
4. Add the chopped garlic into the pan.
5. Add the tomatoes, oregano, bay leaf, salt, black pepper, thyme, smoked paprika, mix spice powder, and chives into the pan.
6. Cook the ingredients well.
7. Add the chickpeas into the mixture.
8. Add the vegetable stock and water into the pan.
9. Mix the soup well.
10. Place a lid on top of the pan.
11. Cook the soup for ten to fifteen minutes.
12. Dish out the soup when the chickpeas are done.

13. Garnish the dish with chopped parsley on top.
14. Your dish is ready to be served.

2.10 Greek Souvlaki Recipe

Preparation Time: 30 minutes
Cooking Time: 10 minutes
Serving: 4

Ingredients:

- Half tablespoon of chopped garlic,
- Three tablespoons of olive oil
- Two tablespoons of granulated sugar
- Two tablespoons of chopped parsley
- One tablespoon of smoked paprika
- Two tablespoons of fresh oregano
- Two tablespoons of fresh thyme
- Half cup of chopped fresh chives
- One teaspoon of mixed spice powder
- Half teaspoon of smoked paprika
- One pound of chicken thighs
- Pita bread

Instructions:
1. Take a large bowl.
2. Add all the ingredients in the bowl.
3. Mix the marinade well.
4. Roast the chicken pieces over a grill pan.
5. Dish out when the chicken pieces are golden brown on both sides.
6. Serve the souvlaki with pita bread on the side.
7. Your dish is ready to be served.

2.11 Greek Beef and Eggplant Lasagna (Moussaka) Recipe

Preparation Time: 30 minutes
Cooking Time: 90 minutes
Serving: 8

Ingredients:

- One tablespoon of minced garlic
- Two tablespoons of fresh chopped dill
- One cup of feta cheese
- Two cups of beef mince
- A pinch of salt
- A pinch of crushed black pepper
- One cup of eggplant pieces
- Two tablespoons of olive oil
- Three cups of baby spinach
- Two cups of russet potatoes
- One cup of chopped onions
- Two cups of tomato sauce
- Two cups of béchamel sauce

Instructions:

1. Take a large bowl.
2. Add the eggplant, beef mince, potatoes, baby spinach into a bowl.
3. Mix the olive oil, salt, and crushed black pepper into the bowl.
4. Bake the ingredients in an oven for about twenty minutes.
5. Take a large pan.
6. Add the olive oil and onion into the pan.
7. Cook the onions until they turn soft.
8. Add the minced garlic into the pan.
9. Cook the ingredients well.
10. Add the feta cheese, salt, and black pepper into the pan.
11. Mix all the ingredients well and add the chopped dill into the pan.
12. Add the baked beef and vegetables into the pan and then mix everything well.
13. Add the tomato sauce and béchamel sauce on top of the vegetable mixture.
14. Bake for another ten minutes.
15. Your dish is ready to be served.

Chapter 3: The Famous Greek Dinner Recipes

Greek dinner recipes are extremely healthy and loved by people everywhere in the world. Following are some classic dinner recipes that are rich in healthy nutrients, and you can easily make them with the detailed instructions list in each recipe:

3.1 Greek Stuffed Grape Leaves Recipe

Preparation Time: 10 minutes
Cooking Time: 20 minutes
Serving: 2

Ingredients:

- Half cup of cooked rice
- One cup of tomato paste
- Two tablespoons of unsalted butter
- Three tablespoons of granulated sugar
- Two cups of cooked beef
- One teaspoon of minced ginger
- Two cups of mixed cheese
- Chopped fresh parsley
- Two tablespoons of olive oil
- One pound of grape leaves
- Two cups of tomatoes
- A pinch of salt
- A pinch of black pepper
- One cup of chopped red onions
- One tablespoon of minced garlic

Instructions:
1. Take a large pan.
2. Add the butter and chopped onions into the pan.
3. Cook the onion until it turns soft.
4. Add the garlic and ginger as well as the beef mince, tomatoes, and tomato paste.

5. Cook the beef well for about ten minutes.
6. Add the granulated sugar, cooked rice, salt and pepper.
7. Mix everything well and dish out.
8. Clean the grape leaves and add the cooked mixture into it.
9. Roll the grape leaves.
10. Add the mixed cheese on top and place the grape leaves on a greased baking tray.
11. Steam the grape leaves for about ten to fifteen minutes.
12. Garnish the grape leaves with freshly chopped parsley leaves.
13. Your dish is ready to be served.

3.2 Greek Baked Orzo Recipe

Preparation Time: 30 minutes
Cooking Time: 30 minutes
Serving: 4

Ingredients:

- One cup of uncooked orzo
- Two cups of chicken pieces
- Eight ounces of freshly cut spinach
- One tablespoon of fresh dill
- Four teaspoons of olive oil
- One teaspoon of dried oregano
- Two cloves of chopped garlic
- Two cups of whole milk
- Five ounces of sun-dried tomatoes
- One cup of crumbled feta cheese
- One teaspoon of lemon pepper
- One teaspoon of salt
- One teaspoon of pepper

Instructions:
1. Take a large bowl.
2. Add the pepper, lemon pepper, fresh dill, dried oregano, and salt into the bowl.
3. Mix all the ingredients well.

4. Add the chicken pieces, orzo, olive oil, and spinach into the bowl.
5. Mix the ingredients well and add the chopped garlic and the rest of the ingredients.
6. Mix all the ingredients of both the bowls together.
7. Pour the mixture into a greased baking dish.
8. Bake the orzo for twenty-five to thirty minutes.
9. Dish out the orzo when done.
10. The dish is ready to be served.

3.3 Greek Spanakopita Recipe

Preparation Time: 40 minutes
Cooking Time: 40 minutes
Serving: 6

Ingredients:

For dough:
- Two cups of all-purpose flour
- Two teaspoons of fine sea salt
- Half cup of unsalted soft butter
- Two whole egg
- A quarter cup of ice water

For filling:
- One cup of feta cheese
- Four eggs
- Half teaspoon of freshly grated nutmeg
- A pinch of salt
- One tablespoon of olive oil
- A quarter cup of chopped onion
- One teaspoon of minced garlic
- One tablespoon of milk
- Half cup of chopped spinach
- A pinch of crushed black pepper

Instructions:
1. Take a large bowl.
2. Add the flour and sea salt into the bowl.
3. Mix the ingredients well and add the eggs, water, and softened butter into the bowl.
4. Mix all the ingredients well to form a dough.
5. Take a large pan.
6. Add the olive oil into the pan.
7. Add the onions and garlic when the oil heats up.
8. Cook the onions until they turn soft.
9. Mix the eggs and add the chopped spinach into the pan.
10. Cook the ingredients until the spinach is wilted.
11. Add the feta cheese, milk, black pepper, salt, and freshly grated nutmeg into the pan.

12. Cook the ingredients for about five minutes.
13. Switch off the stove and let the mixture cool down.
14. Roll out the dough and lay half of it in a round baking dish.
15. Add the cooked mixture to the dough and cover the mixture with the rest of the dough.
16. Bake the spanakopita for about twenty to twenty-five minutes.
17. Dish out the spanakopita when it is done.
18. Your dish is ready to be served.

3.4 Greek Cheese Pies (Tiropita) Recipe

Preparation Time: 30 minutes
Cooking Time: 50 minutes
Serving: 4

Ingredients:

- A quarter cup of Greek feta cheese
- One cup of gruyere cheese
- One cup of milk
- Four whole eggs
- A quarter cup of Philadelphia cheese
- half cup of Melted butter
- One pack of organic phyllo sheets
- One sprig of fresh thyme leaves
- Two tablespoons of sesame seeds
- A pinch of salt
- A pinch of freshly crushed black pepper

Instructions:
1. Take a large pan.
2. Add the butter into the pan and melt it.
3. Add the sesame seeds, eggs, salt, and pepper into the pan.
4. Cook the eggs well, and then add the thyme into the pan.
5. Cook the dish for two to three minutes and then dish out.
6. Add the milk, Philadelphia cheese, Greek feta cheese, and gruyere cheese when the mixture cools down.

7. Mix everything well.
8. Cut the phyllo sheets in the desired shape and add the above mixture into the middle.
9. Place the pies on a greased baking tray.
10. Place the baking tray in a preheated oven.
11. Bake the pies for about forty-five to fifty minutes.
12. Dish out the pies when they attain a golden brown color.
13. The dish is ready to be served.

3.5 Greek Slow Cooked Lamb Gyros Recipe

Preparation Time: 10 minutes
Cooking Time: 30 minutes
Serving: 4

Ingredients:

- Four flatbreads
- Half cup of vegetable broth
- A quarter cup of lemon juice
- One cup of tzatziki sauce
- Half cup of sliced red onion
- Half cup of sliced tomatoes
- Half cup of romaine lettuce
- One tablespoon of minced garlic
- One cup of tomato paste
- Two tablespoons of olive oil
- One tablespoon of garlic powder
- One tablespoon of dried thyme
- Half teaspoon of ground cinnamon
- Two tablespoons of chili powder
- A quarter teaspoon of fresh nutmeg
- A pinch of sea salt
- Two cups of lamb pieces

Instructions:
1. Take a large pan.
2. Add the olive oil and garlic into the pan.
3. Add the oregano, tomato paste, smoked paprika, nutmeg, chili powder, thyme, and salt.
4. Add the vegetable broth, lemon juice, and lamb pieces into the pan.
5. Slow down the stove and cook for about thirty minutes.
6. Cook the ingredients well for about fifteen minutes.
7. Bake the flatbreads for about two to three minutes.
8. Cut the flatbreads in between to form a pouch structure.
9. Add the cooked mixture into the flatbread and line it with tzatziki sauce, romaine lettuce, sliced tomatoes, and red onions.
10. Your dish is ready to be served.

3.6 Greek Lamb Stuffed Courgettes Recipe

Preparation Time: 10 minutes
Cooking Time: 20 minutes
Serving: 2

Ingredients:

- Four tablespoons of olive oil
- One cup of chopped onion
- One teaspoon of cinnamon
- Four chopped garlic
- A quarter cup of raisins
- Six courgettes
- Two cups of lamb mince
- A quarter cup of chopped raisins
- Two tablespoons of pine nuts
- One cup feta cheese
- Chopped mint leaves

Instructions:

1. Take a pan.
2. Add oil into the pan.
3. Add all the ingredients except the mint, feta cheese, and courgettes into the pan.
4. Cook the ingredients well and then grind them.
5. Add the paste on top of the courgettes and cover it with feta cheese.
6. Bake the courgettes for about ten to fifteen minutes.
7. Dish out the courgettes and garnish them with chopped mint leaves.
8. Your dish is ready to be served.

3.7 Greek Lamb Kleftiko Recipe

Preparation Time: 30 minutes
Cooking Time: 30 minutes
Serving: 4

Ingredients:

- Two cups of lamb pieces
- One tablespoon of fresh dill
- Four teaspoons of olive oil
- One teaspoon of dried oregano
- Two cloves of chopped garlic
- Two cups of whole milk
- Five ounces of sun-dried tomatoes
- One cup of crumbled feta cheese
- One teaspoon of lemon pepper
- One teaspoon of salt
- One teaspoon of pepper

Instructions:

1. Take a large bowl.
2. Add the pepper, lemon pepper, fresh dill, dried oregano, and salt into the bowl.
3. Mix all the ingredients well.
4. Add the lamb pieces and olive oil to the bowl.
5. Mix the ingredients well and add the chopped garlic and the rest of the ingredients.
6. Mix all the ingredients of both the bowls together.
7. Add the mixture to a greased baking dish.
8. Bake the lamb kleftiko for twenty-five to thirty minutes.
9. Dish out the kleftiko when done.
10. The dish is ready to be served.

3.8 Greek Spiced Lamb Cutlets with Smoked Aubergine Recipe

Preparation Time: 30 minutes
Cooking Time: 30 minutes
Serving: 4

Ingredients:

- Two cups of lamb pieces
- One tablespoon of fresh dill
- Four teaspoons of olive oil
- One teaspoon of dried oregano
- Two teaspoons of mixed spice
- Two cloves of chopped garlic
- Two cups of aubergine
- One cup of crumbled feta cheese
- One teaspoon of lemon pepper
- One teaspoon of salt
- One teaspoon of pepper

Instructions:

1. Take a large bowl.
2. Add the pepper, aubergine pieces, mixed spice, lemon pepper, fresh dill, dried oregano, and salt into the bowl.
3. Mix all the ingredients well.
4. Add the lamb pieces and olive oil to the bowl.
5. Mix the ingredients well and add the chopped garlic and the rest of the ingredients.
6. Mix all the ingredients of both the bowls together.
7. Add the mixture to a greased baking dish.
8. Grill the lamb and aubergine for twenty-five to thirty minutes.
9. Dish out the lamb and aubergine when done.
10. The dish is ready to be served.

3.9 Greek Aborigine and Lamb Pasticcio Recipe

Preparation Time: 30 minutes
Cooking Time: 90 minutes
Serving: 8

Ingredients:

- One tablespoon of minced garlic
- Two tablespoons of fresh chopped dill
- One cup of feta cheese
- Two cups of lamb mince
- A pinch of salt
- A pinch of crushed black pepper
- One cup of aubergine pieces
- Two tablespoons of olive oil
- Three cups of baby spinach
- Two cups of russet potatoes
- One cup of chopped onions
- Two cups of tomato sauce
- Two cups of béchamel sauce

Instructions:

1. Take a large bowl.
2. Add the aubergine, lamb mince, potatoes, baby spinach into a bowl.
3. Mix the olive oil, salt, and crushed black pepper into the bowl.
4. Bake the ingredients in an oven for about twenty minutes.
5. Take a large pan.
6. Add the olive oil and onion into the pan.
7. Cook the onions until they turn soft.
8. Add the minced garlic into the pan.
9. Cook the ingredients well.
10. Add the feta cheese, salt, and black pepper into the pan.
11. Mix all the ingredients well and add the chopped dill into the pan.
12. Add the baked lamb and vegetables into the pan and then mix everything well.
13. Add the tomato sauce and béchamel sauce on top of the vegetable mixture.
14. Bake for another ten minutes.
15. Your dish is ready to be served.

3.10 Greek Green Salad with Marinated Feta Recipe

Preparation Time: 20 minutes
Cooking Time: 15 minutes
Serving: 2

Ingredients:

For the dressing:
- Half teaspoon of kosher salt
- Two teaspoons of freshly ground black pepper
- A quarter cup of red wine vinegar
- Half cup of olive oil
- Two tablespoons of minced garlic
- Two teaspoons of fresh oregano
- Half teaspoon of dried oregano

For salad:
- One cup of marinated feta cheese
- Half pound of bread slices
- Half teaspoon of minced garlic
- Two tablespoons of olive oil
- Half cup of Kalamata olives
- One cup of red-orange bell pepper
- One cup of English cucumber
- One cup of cherry tomatoes

Instructions:
1. Take a small bowl.
2. Add the olive oil and minced garlic into it.
3. Mix it well and spread it on the bread slices.
4. Dish out the bread slices when they are done.
5. Take a large bowl.
6. Add the English cucumber, Kalamata olives, red-orange bell pepper, cherry tomatoes, and marinated feta cheese into the bowl.
7. Mix everything well and set it aside.
8. Take a small bowl.
9. Add the olive oil, red wine vinegar, kosher salt, minced garlic, freshly crushed black pepper, fresh oregano, and dried oregano.
10. Mix everything well.

11. Pour this dressing on the prepared salad.
12. Mix everything well and add the toasted bread slices to the side.
13. Your dish is ready to be served.

3.11 Greek Lamb Pitas Recipe

Preparation Time: 10 minutes
Cooking Time: 15 minutes
Serving: 2

Ingredients:

- Two tablespoons of olive oil
- Two slices of pita bread
- Two large eggs
- One ripe cherry tomato
- Two cups of lamb pieces
- One cup of chopped onion
- Half cup of chopped basil
- A quarter cup of crumbled feta cheese
- A pinch of salt
- A pinch of black pepper
- A bunch of chopped cilantro

Instructions:

1. Take a large pan.
2. Add the olive oil into the pan.
3. Add the onion and salt into the pan.
4. Cook the onions well and then add the black pepper into the pan.
5. Add the lamb pieces into the mixture.
6. Add the chopped basil into the mixture.
7. Cook the ingredients well for about fifteen minutes.
8. Dish out when the lamb pieces are done.
9. Let the meat cool down and then add the crumbled feta cheese into it.
10. Mix well.
11. Heat the pita breads.
12. Cut a hole into the bread and add the cooked mixture into it.
13. Garnish the bread with chopped cilantro.
14. Your dish is ready to be served.

Chapter 4: The Famous Greek Dessert Recipes

You should really try Greek desserts if you are a sweet tooth. Following are some yummy dessert recipes that are rich in healthy nutrients:

4.1 Greek Butter Cookies Recipe

Preparation Time: 20 minutes
Cooking Time: 20 minutes
Serving: 4

Ingredients:

- Half teaspoon of nutmeg
- One teaspoon of vanilla extract
- Three and a half cups of flour
- Half cup of sugar
- A cup of salted butter
- One tablespoon of yeast
- Two large eggs
- Half teaspoon of kosher salt

Instructions:

1. Take a large bowl.
2. Add the dry ingredients in a bowl.
3. Mix all the ingredients well.
4. Add the white sugar and yeast in a bowl with two tablespoons of hot water.
5. Place the yeast mixture in a damp place.
6. Add the butter into the wet ingredients.
7. Add the yeast mixture and eggs into the cookie mixture.
8. Add the formed mixture into a piping bag.
9. Make small round cookies on a baking dish and bake the cookies.
10. Dish out the cookies when done.
11. The dish is ready to be served.

4.2 Greek Honey Cookies Recipe

Preparation Time: 20 minutes
Cooking Time: 20 minutes
Serving: 4

Ingredients:

- Half teaspoon of nutmeg
- One teaspoon of vanilla extract
- Three and a half cups of flour
- Half cup of honey
- Half cup of oil
- One tablespoon of yeast
- Two large eggs
- Half teaspoon of kosher salt

Instructions:
1. Take a large bowl.
2. Add the dry ingredients in a bowl.
3. Mix all the ingredients well.
4. Add the honey and yeast in a bowl with two tablespoons of hot water.
5. Place the yeast mixture in a damp place.
6. Add the oil into the wet ingredients.
7. Add the yeast mixture and eggs into the cookie mixture.
8. Add the formed mixture into a piping bag.
9. Make small round cookies on a baking dish and bake the cookies.
10. Dish out the cookies when done.
11. The dish is ready to be served.

4.3 Greek Walnut Cake Recipe

Preparation Time: 30 minutes
Cooking Time: 25 minutes
Serving: 4

Ingredients:

- One cup of vanilla sauce
- Half cup of butter
- A quarter cup of sugar
- A quarter teaspoon of ground cardamom
- A cup of flour
- A pinch of baking soda,
- One egg
- A cup of sliced almonds

For Frosting

- Half cup of vanilla sauce
- Half cup of heavy cream
- Half cup of butter
- Half cup of brown sugar
- A quarter teaspoon of cinnamon

Instructions:

1. Take a large bowl.
2. Add the cake batter and mix all the ingredients.
3. Make the batter and pour it into a baking dish.
4. Make sure the baking dish is properly greased and lined with parchment paper.
5. Add the walnut mixture and mix up all the ingredients.
6. Bake the cake.
7. Dish it out when done.
8. Make the vanilla and cream frosting by first beating the butter and cream until they turn fluffy.
9. Add in the rest of the ingredients and beat for five minutes.
10. Add the vanilla and cream frosting on top of the cake.
11. Make sure to cover all the sides of the cake with frosting.
12. Cut the cake into slices.
13. The dish is ready to be served.

4.4 Greek Baklava Recipe

Preparation Time: 20 minutes
Cooking Time: 40 minutes
Serving: 4

Ingredients:

- Eight ounces of butter
- A pack of phyllo sheets
- A teaspoon of vanilla extract
- Half cup of chopped nuts (of your choice)
- A cup of honey
- A cup of sugar
- A teaspoon of ground cinnamon
- A cup of water

Instructions:

1. Take a large bowl.
2. Add the butter into it and beat well.
3. Add the nuts, cinnamon and honey into the butter bowl.
4. Mix the ingredients well.
5. Add the dried mint into the bowl and mix well.
6. Spread the phyllo sheets in a greased baking tray.
7. Add the nut mixture into the phyllo sheets and cover it with more phyllo sheets.
8. Bake the baklava for about forty minutes.
9. Add sugar and water in a saucepan and cook.
10. Dis out the baklava and cut it into pieces.
11. Pour the sugar syrup on top of the baklava
12. Dish out the baklava.
13. The dish is ready to be served.

4.5 Greek Orange Cake Recipe

Preparation Time: 30 minutes
Cooking Time: 25 minutes
Serving: 4

Ingredients:

- A cup of orange juice
- Half cup of butter
- A quarter cup of sugar
- A quarter teaspoon ground cardamom
- A cup of flour
- A pinch of baking soda,
- An egg
- Two teaspoon of orange zest

Instructions:

1. Take a large bowl.
2. Add the cake batter and mix all the ingredients.
3. Make the batter and pour it into a baking dish.
4. Make sure the baking dish is properly greased and lined with parchment paper.
5. Bake the cake.
6. Dish it out when done.
7. Cut the cake into slices.
8. The dish is ready to be served.

4.6 Greek Donuts (Loukoumades) Recipe

Preparation Time: 10 minutes
Cooking Time: 30 minutes
Serving: 6

Ingredients:

- Half cup of butter
- Eight eggs
- Two cups of sugar
- Three cups of flour

- A cup of milk
- A tablespoon of baking powder
- Two tablespoons of sour cream
- A teaspoon of cardamom sugar
- A teaspoon of baking soda
- Two tablespoons of honey

Instructions:
1. In a large bowl, mix all the ingredients except the cardamom sugar and honey.
2. Form semi-thick dough from the mixture.
3. Heat a pan full of oil.
4. Make a round doughnut-like structure with the help of a doughnut cutter.
5. Fry the doughnuts.
6. Let the doughnuts cool down.
7. Drizzle the honey on top of the doughnuts.
8. Add the cinnamon sugar all over the doughnuts.
9. Your dish is ready to be served.

4.7 Greek Milk Custard Pudding Recipe

Preparation Time: 20 minutes
Cooking Time: 30 minutes
Serving: 4

Ingredients:

- Two cups of whole milk
- Two cups of water
- Four tablespoon of cornstarch
- Four tablespoon of white sugar
- Two egg yolks
- A quarter teaspoon of cinnamon powder

Instructions:
1. Take a large saucepan.
2. Add the water and whole milk.
3. Let the liquid boil for five minutes.
4. Add the egg yolks and sugar into the milk mixture.
5. Cook all the ingredients well for thirty minutes or until it starts to get thick.

6. Keep stirring continuously.
7. Add the cinnamon powder on top.
8. The dish is ready to be served.

4.8 Greek Almond Syrup Pastries Recipe

Preparation Time: 20 minutes
Cooking Time: 40 minutes
Serving: 4

Ingredients:

- Eight ounces of almond syrup
- A pack of phyllo sheets
- A teaspoon of dried nutmeg
- Half cup of chopped nuts (of your choice)
- A cup of honey thyme
- Seven ounces of butter

Instructions:

1. Take a large bowl.
2. Add the butter into it and beat well.
3. Add the nuts and almond syrup into the butter bowl.
4. Mix the ingredients well.
5. Spread the phyllo sheets in a greased baking tray.
6. Add the nut mixture into the phyllo sheets and cover it with more phyllo sheets.
7. Bake the pastry for about forty minutes.
8. Dish out the pastry.
9. Drizzle the honey thyme on top of the pie.
10. The dish is ready to be served.

4.9 Greek Almond Shortbread Recipe

Preparation Time: 10 minutes
Cooking Time: 40 minutes
Serving: 4

Ingredients:

- Half teaspoon of vanilla bean paste
- Two and a half cups flour
- Half teaspoon baking powder
- A cup of unsalted butter
- An egg yolk

- Two cups icing sugar
- Half cup chopped almonds

Instructions:
1. Take a large bowl.
2. Add the vanilla bean paste, flour, baking powder, unsalted butter, egg yolk, and almonds into the bowl.
3. Mix all the ingredients and add them to a baking tray.
4. Bake the mixture for thirty minutes.
5. Dish out the bread and cut it into slices.
6. Dust the bread with icing sugar.
7. Your dish is ready to be served.

4.10 Greek Orange Blossom Baklava Recipe

Preparation Time: 20 minutes
Cooking Time: 40 minutes
Serving: 4

Ingredients:

- Eight ounces of butter
- A pack of phyllo sheets
- A teaspoon of vanilla extract
- Half cup of chopped nuts (of your choice)
- A cup of honey
- A cup of sugar
- A teaspoon of a ground orange powder
- A cup of water

Instructions:
1. Take a large bowl.
2. Add the butter into it and beat well.
3. Add the nuts, orange powder, and honey into the butter bowl.
4. Mix the ingredients well.
5. Add the dried mint into the bowl and mix well.
6. Spread the phyllo sheets in a greased baking tray.
7. Add the nut mixture into the phyllo sheets and cover it with more phyllo sheets.

8. Bake the baklava for about forty minutes.
9. Add sugar and water to a saucepan and cook.
10. Dish out the baklava and cut it into pieces.
11. Pour the sugar syrup on top of the baklava
12. Dish out the baklava.
13. The dish is ready to be served.

4.11 Greek Honey and Rosewater Baklava Recipe

Preparation Time: 20 minutes
Cooking Time: 40 minutes
Serving: 4

Ingredients:

- Eight ounces of butter
- A pack of phyllo sheets
- A teaspoon of vanilla extract
- Half cup of chopped nuts (of your choice)
- A cup of honey
- A cup of sugar
- A teaspoon of rose water
- A cup of water

Instructions:
1. Take a large bowl.
2. Add the butter into it and beat well.
3. Add the nuts, rose water, and honey into the butter bowl.
4. Mix the ingredients well.
5. Add the dried mint into the bowl and mix well.
6. Spread the phyllo sheets in a greased baking tray.
7. Add the nut mixture into the phyllo sheets and cover it with more phyllo sheets.
8. Bake the baklava for about forty minutes.
9. Add sugar and water in a saucepan and cook.
10. Dish out the baklava and cut it into pieces.
11. Pour the sugar syrup on top of the baklava
12. Dish out the baklava.
13. The dish is ready to be served.

Chapter 5: The Famous Greek Snack Recipes

Greek snacks are famous all around the world. Following are some amazing Greek snack recipes that are rich in healthy nutrients, and you can easily make them with the detailed instructions list in each recipe:

5.1 Greek Tzatziki Dip Recipe

Preparation Time: 30 minutes
Cooking Time: 15 minutes
Serving: 4

Ingredients:

- One and a half cups of Greek yoghurt
- One tablespoon of chopped fresh dill
- Half chopped cucumber
- Two tablespoons of olive oil
- Half teaspoon of salt
- Two teaspoons of minced garlic
- One tablespoon of white vinegar

Instructions:
1. Take a large bowl.
2. Add all the dried ingredients into the bowl.
3. Mix well and refrigerate for ten minutes.
4. Add the wet ingredients into the bowl.
5. Mix well.
6. Your dish is ready to be served.

5.2 Greek Fried Cheese Recipe

Preparation Time: 40 minutes
Cooking Time: 30 minutes
Serving: 4

Ingredients:

- One pound hard cheese
- Vegetable oil
- One cup all-purpose flour

Instructions:

1. Cut the cheese into slices.
2. Dip it in all-purpose flour.
3. Take a large frying pan.
4. Add oil into the pan and heat well.
5. Add the cheese slices and deep fry until they turn golden brown.
6. Your dish is ready to be served.

5.3 Greek Fries Recipe

Preparation Time: 40 minutes
Cooking Time: 30 minutes
Serving: 4

Ingredients:

- One pound russet potatoes
- Vegetable oil
- One cup all-purpose flour
- One cup crumbled feta cheese
- One cup salsa

Instructions:

1. Cut the potatoes into sticks.
2. Dip it in all-purpose flour.
3. Take a large frying pan.
4. Add oil into the pan and heat well.

5. Add the potato sticks and deep fry until they turn golden brown.
6. Dish out the fries and add the salsa and feta cheese on top.
7. Your dish is ready to be served.

5.4 Greek Feta Dip Recipe

Preparation Time: 30 minutes
Cooking Time: 15 minutes
Serving: 4

Ingredients:

- One and a half cups of Greek yoghurt
- One tablespoon of chopped fresh dill
- Half chopped feta cheese
- Two tablespoons of olive oil
- Half teaspoon of salt
- Two teaspoons of minced garlic
- One tablespoon of white vinegar

Instructions:
1. Take a large bowl.
2. Add all the dried ingredients into the bowl.
3. Mix well and refrigerate for ten minutes.
4. Add the wet ingredients into the bowl.
5. Mix well.
6. Your dish is ready to be served.

5.5 Greek Eggplant Dip Recipe

Preparation Time: 30 minutes
Cooking Time: 15 minutes
Serving: 4

Ingredients:

- One and a half cups of Greek yoghurt
- One tablespoon of chopped fresh dill
- Half chopped roasted eggplant
- Two tablespoons of olive oil

- Half teaspoon of salt
- Two teaspoons of minced garlic

Instructions:
1. Take a large bowl.
2. Add all the ingredients and mix well.
3. Garnish the dish with fresh dill.
4. Your dish is ready to be served.

5.6 Greek Spanakopita Spring Rolls Recipe

Preparation Time: 40 minutes
Cooking Time: 40 minutes
Serving: 6

Ingredients:

- One pack of spring roll wrappers
- Vegetable oil

For filling:
- One cup of feta cheese
- Four eggs
- Half teaspoon of freshly grated nutmeg
- A pinch of salt
- One tablespoon of olive oil
- A quarter cup of chopped onion
- One teaspoon of minced garlic
- One tablespoon of milk
- Half cup of chopped spinach
- A pinch of crushed black pepper

Instructions:
1. Take a large pan.
2. Add the olive oil into the pan.
3. Add the onions and garlic when the oil heats up.
4. Cook the onions until they turn soft.
5. Mix the eggs and add the chopped spinach into the pan.
6. Cook the ingredients until the spinach is wilted.

7. Add the feta cheese, milk, black pepper, salt, and freshly grated nutmeg into the pan.
8. Cook the ingredients for about five minutes.
9. Switch off the stove and let the mixture cool down.
10. Add the mixture on the spring roll wrappers and roll it.
11. Deep fry the spring rolls until they turn golden brown.
12. Dish out the spanakopita when it is done.
13. Your dish is ready to be served.

5.7 Greek Tortilla Pinwheels Recipe

Preparation Time: 40 minutes
Cooking Time: 40 minutes
Serving: 6

Ingredients:

- One pack of tortillas
- Vegetable oil

For filling:
- One cup of feta cheese
- One pound beef mince
- Half teaspoon of freshly grated nutmeg
- A pinch of salt
- One tablespoon of olive oil
- A quarter cup of chopped onion
- One teaspoon of minced garlic
- One tablespoon of milk
- Half cup of chopped spinach
- A pinch of crushed black pepper

Instructions:

1. Take a large pan.
2. Add the olive oil into the pan.
3. Add the onions and garlic when the oil heats up.
4. Cook the onions until they turn soft.
5. Mix the beef and add the chopped spinach into the pan.
6. Cook the ingredients until the spinach is wilted.
7. Add the feta cheese, milk, black pepper, salt, and freshly grated nutmeg into the pan.
8. Cook the ingredients for about five minutes.
9. Switch off the stove and let the mixture cool down.
10. Add the mixture on the tortillas and roll it.
11. Bake the pinwheels until they turn golden brown.
12. Dish out the pinwheels when they are done.
13. Your dish is ready to be served.

5.8 Greek Stuffed Cucumber Bites Recipe

Preparation Time: 40 minutes
Cooking Time: 40 minutes
Serving: 6

Ingredients:

- One pound cucumber

For filling:

- One cup of feta cheese
- One pound chicken mince
- Half teaspoon of freshly grated nutmeg
- A pinch of salt
- One tablespoon of olive oil
- A quarter cup of chopped onion
- One teaspoon of minced garlic
- A pinch of crushed black pepper
- Fresh mint

Instructions:

1. Take a large pan.
2. Add the olive oil into the pan.
3. Add the onions and garlic when the oil heats up.
4. Cook the onions until they turn soft.
5. Mix the chicken into the pan.
6. Add the feta cheese, black pepper, salt, and freshly grated nutmeg into the pan.
7. Cook the ingredients for about five minutes.
8. Switch off the stove and let the mixture cool down.
9. Add the mixture on the cucumber pieces.
10. Garnish the dish with chopped mint leaves.
11. Your dish is ready to be served.

5.9 Greek Salad Cracker Recipe

Preparation Time: 20 minutes
Cooking Time: 15 minutes
Serving: 2

Ingredients:

For the dressing:
- Half teaspoon of kosher salt
- Two teaspoons of freshly ground black pepper
- A quarter cup of red wine vinegar
- Half cup of olive oil
- Two tablespoons of minced garlic
- Two teaspoons of fresh oregano
- Half teaspoon of dried oregano

For salad:
- One cup of feta cheese
- Half pound of crispbread slices
- Half teaspoon of minced garlic
- Two tablespoons of olive oil
- Half cup of Kalamata olives
- One cup of red-orange bell pepper
- One cup of English cucumber
- One cup of cherry tomatoes

Instructions:
1. Take a small bowl.
2. Add the olive oil and minced garlic into it.
3. Mix in the bread slices.
4. Bake the slices for ten minutes.
5. Dish out the bread slices when they are done.
6. Take a large bowl.
7. Add the English cucumber, Kalamata olives, red-orange bell pepper, cherry tomatoes, and feta cheese into the bowl.
8. Mix everything well and set it aside.
9. Take a small bowl.
10. Add the olive oil, red wine vinegar, kosher salt, minced garlic, freshly crushed black pepper, fresh oregano, and dried oregano.
11. Mix everything well.

12. Pour this dressing on the prepared salad.
13. Mix everything well and add it on top of the toasted bread slices.
14. Your dish is ready to be served.

5.10 Greek Pita Bread Bites Recipe

Preparation Time: 40 minutes
Cooking Time: 30 minutes
Serving: 4

Ingredients:

- One pound pita bread bites
- Vegetable oil
- One cup all-purpose flour
- One cup crumbled feta cheese
- One cup salsa

Instructions:

1. Cut the pita bread into bite-size pieces.
2. Dip it in all-purpose flour.
3. Take a large frying pan.
4. Add oil into the pan and heat well.
5. Add the pita bread and deep fry until they turn golden brown.
6. Dish out the bread and add the salsa and feta cheese on top.
7. Your dish is ready to be served.

5.11 Greek Zucchini Balls (Kolokithokeftedes) Recipe

Preparation Time: 10 minutes
Cooking Time: 20 minutes
Serving: 2

Ingredients:

- One chopped red onion
- Two minced garlic cloves
- A pinch of salt
- A pinch of black pepper
- Half cup of mint leaves
- Two cups of grated zucchini

- Half teaspoon of oregano
- One egg
- Two tablespoons of olive oil
- One cup of Greek yoghurt

Instructions:
1. Take a large bowl.
2. Add the grated zucchini, spices, mint, onion, garlic, and egg into the bowl.
3. Mix all the ingredients well and form round ball structures.
4. Fry the zucchini balls in olive oil until they turn golden brown.
5. Dish out the balls.
6. Serve the zucchini balls with Greek yoghurt on the side.
7. Your dish is ready to be served.

Chapter 6: The Famous Greek Vegetarian Recipes

Greek vegetarian dishes are extremely wondrous and loveable. Following are some amazing Greek vegetarian recipes that are rich in healthy nutrients, and you can easily make them with the detailed instructions list in each recipe.

6.1 Greek Jackfruit Gyros Recipe

Preparation Time: 10 minutes
Cooking Time: 30 minutes
Serving: 4

Ingredients:

- Four flatbreads
- Half cup of vegetable broth
- A quarter cup of lemon juice
- One cup of tzatziki sauce
- Half cup of sliced red onion
- Half cup of sliced tomatoes
- Half cup of romaine lettuce
- One tablespoon of minced garlic
- One cup of tomato paste
- Two tablespoons of olive oil
- One tablespoon of garlic powder
- One tablespoon of dried thyme
- Half teaspoon of ground cinnamon
- Two tablespoons of chili powder
- A quarter teaspoon of fresh nutmeg
- A pinch of sea salt
- Two cups of jackfruit pieces

Instructions:
1. Take a large pan.
2. Add the olive oil and garlic into the pan.
3. Add the oregano, tomato paste, smoked paprika, nutmeg, chili powder, thyme, and salt.
4. Add the vegetable broth, lemon juice, and jackfruit pieces into the pan.
5. Cook the ingredients well for about five minutes.
6. Bake the flatbreads for about two to three minutes.

7. Cut the flatbreads in between to form a pouch structure.
8. Add the cooked mixture into the flatbread and line it with tzatziki sauce, romaine lettuce, sliced tomatoes, and red onions.
9. Your dish is ready to be served.

6.2 Greek Vegan Skordalia Recipe

Preparation Time: 40 minutes
Cooking Time: 30 minutes
Serving: 4

Ingredients:

- A quarter cup almond meal
- Half cup olive oil
- One russet potato
- Two tablespoons lemon juice
- Two teaspoons red wine vinegar
- Ten cloves of chopped garlic
- Half teaspoon of salt

Instructions:
1. Take a saucepan.
2. Boil the potatoes in the saucepan.
3. Drain the potatoes when done.
4. Mash the potatoes.
5. Add the garlic, lemon juice, almond meal, salt, red wine vinegar, and olive oil into the mashed potatoes.
6. Mix everything well.
7. Your dish is ready to be served.

6.3 Greek Orzo Pasta Salad with Vegan Feta Recipe

Preparation Time: 30 minutes
Cooking Time: 20 minutes
Serving: 4

Ingredients:

- One chopped red onion

- Eight ounces of orzo pasta
- Half cup of Kalamata olives
- Two cups of cherry tomatoes
- Half cup of chopped parsley
- Two cups of vegan cheese
- One chopped cucumber
- One cup of lemon dressing

Instructions:
1. Take a saucepan and add the water in it.
2. Boil the water and add the orzo pasta into it.
3. Drain the orzo pasta when done.
4. Add the rest of the ingredients into the pasta.
5. Mix everything well.
6. Your dish is ready to be served.

6.4 Greek Chickpea Gyros Recipe

Preparation Time: 10 minutes
Cooking Time: 30 minutes
Serving: 4

Ingredients:

- Four flatbreads
- Half cup of vegetable broth
- A quarter cup of lemon juice
- One cup of tzatziki sauce
- Half cup of sliced red onion
- Half cup of sliced tomatoes
- Half cup of romaine lettuce
- One tablespoon of minced garlic
- One cup of tomato paste
- Two tablespoons of olive oil
- One tablespoon of garlic powder
- One tablespoon of dried thyme
- Half teaspoon of ground cinnamon
- Two tablespoons of chili powder
- A quarter teaspoon of fresh nutmeg

- A pinch of sea salt
- Two cups of chickpea pieces

Instructions:
1. Take a large pan.
2. Add the olive oil and garlic into the pan.
3. Add the oregano, tomato paste, smoked paprika, nutmeg, chili powder, thyme, and salt.
4. Add the vegetable broth, lemon juice, and chickpea pieces into the pan.
5. Cook the ingredients well for about twenty minutes.
6. Bake the flatbreads for about two to three minutes.
7. Cut the flatbreads in between to form a pouch structure.
8. Add the cooked mixture into the flatbread and line it with tzatziki sauce, romaine lettuce, sliced tomatoes, and red onions.
9. Your dish is ready to be served.

6.5 Greek Vegetarian Moussaka Recipe

Preparation Time: 30 minutes
Cooking Time: 90 minutes
Serving: 8

Ingredients:

- One tablespoon of minced garlic
- Two tablespoons of fresh chopped dill
- One cup of feta cheese
- Two cups of zucchini pieces
- A pinch of salt
- A pinch of crushed black pepper
- One cup of eggplant pieces
- Two tablespoons of olive oil
- Three cups of baby spinach
- Two cups of russet potatoes
- One cup of chopped onions
- Two cups of tomato sauce
- Two cups of béchamel sauce

Instructions:

1. Take a large bowl.
2. Add the eggplant, zucchini pieces, potatoes, baby spinach into a bowl.
3. Mix the olive oil, salt, and crushed black pepper into the bowl.
4. Bake the ingredients in an oven for about twenty minutes.
5. Take a large pan.
6. Add the olive oil and onion into the pan.
7. Cook the onions until they turn soft.
8. Add the minced garlic into the pan.
9. Cook the ingredients well.
10. Add the feta cheese, salt, and black pepper into the pan.
11. Mix all the ingredients well and add the chopped dill into the pan.
12. Add the baked vegetables into the pan and then mix everything well.
13. Add the tomato sauce and béchamel sauce on top of the vegetable mixture.
14. Bake for another ten minutes.
15. Your dish is ready to be served.

6.6 Greek Baked Zucchini and Potatoes Recipe

Preparation Time: 30 minutes
Cooking Time: 30 minutes
Serving: 4

Ingredients:

- Half cup of chopped parsley
- Two tablespoons of oregano leaves
- One tablespoon of rosemary leaves
- Two tablespoons of parsley leaves
- Half cup of chopped onion
- Two tablespoons of olive oil
- Half cup of basil leaves
- One cup of red bell pepper
- One tablespoon of crushed red pepper
- Half teaspoon of fennel leaves
- A pinch of kosher salt
- A pinch of black pepper
- One cup of eggplant pieces
- One cup of zucchini pieces
- One cup of chopped chives
- One cup of cherry tomatoes

- Half cup of savory summer sprigs
- Two tablespoons of minced garlic
- Two tablespoons of dried thyme

Instructions:
1. Take a large pan.
2. Add the olive oil and chopped onions into it.
3. Cook the onions until they turn light brown in color.
4. Add the minced garlic into the pan.
5. Cook the mixture for five minutes.
6. Season the mixture with salt and pepper.
7. Add the spices and all the vegetables.
8. In a bowl, crush the cherry tomatoes and add the salt.
9. Dish the mixture out in a plate when the vegetables are done.
10. Add the crushed tomatoes into the pan.
11. Cook the tomatoes for ten minutes or until they turn soft.
12. Add the vegetable mixture into the pan again.
13. Add the rest of the ingredients into the pan and bake it for about fifteen minutes.
14. Your dish is ready to be served.

6.7 Greek Vegetarian Rice Recipe

Preparation Time: 10 minutes
Cooking Time: 20 minutes
Serving: 2

Ingredients:

- Three cups of chopped mixed vegetables
- Two teaspoons of lemon juice
- Half cup of chopped onions
- Two tablespoons of minced garlic
- Two tablespoons of olive oil
- A pinch of salt
- A pinch of black pepper
- A quarter cup of dried mint
- Two tablespoons of chopped fresh dill
- Two pounds of rice grains
- Two cups of tomato paste
- Two cups of water

Instructions:

1. Take a large saucepan.
2. Add the water into the pan and season it with salt.
3. Boil the water and then add the rice into the water.
4. Boil the rice and then drain it.
5. Take a large pan.
6. Add the olive oil and heat it well.
7. Add the chopped onions into the pan and cook it until it turns soft and fragrant.
8. Add the chopped garlic into the pan.
9. Add the vegetables, tomato paste, lemon juice, salt, and crushed black pepper into the pan.
10. Cook the ingredients for about ten minutes.
11. Add the boiled rice into the pan and mix well.
12. Add the dried mint and chopped dill into the pan.
13. Place a lid on top of the pan.
14. Cook the rice for about five minutes on low heat.
15. Your dish is ready to be served.

6.8 Greek Gigantes Plaki Recipe

Preparation Time: 5 minutes
Cooking Time: 135 minutes
Serving: 4

Ingredients:

- Four tablespoons of finely chopped celery
- Half cup of hot water
- Two cups of finely chopped tomatoes
- One teaspoon of dried oregano leaves
- A pinch of freshly crushed black pepper
- A pinch of kosher salt
- Half cup of olive oil
- Two tablespoons of minced garlic
- Two cups of gigantes plaki
- Half cup of chopped onion
- Four tablespoons of finely chopped parsley

Instructions:

1. Take a pan.
2. Add in the olive oil and onions.
3. Cook the onions until they become soft and fragrant.
4. Add the chopped garlic into the pan.
5. Cook the mixture and add the tomatoes into it.
6. Cover the dish with a lid.
7. Cook the tomatoes until they turn soft.
8. Add the beans into the pan.
9. Cook for five minutes.
10. Add the water, salt, and black pepper into the pan.
11. Mix the ingredients carefully and cover the pan.
12. When the beans are cooked, dish them out.
13. Garnish the dish with chopped celery and parsley leaves on top.
14. Your dish is ready to be served.

6.9 Greek Tomato Fritters Recipe

Preparation Time: 30 minutes
Cooking Time: 30 minutes
Serving: 4

Ingredients:

- One cup of chopped tomatoes
- One cup of red onions
- One cup of gram flour
- A pinch of salt
- Two tablespoons of mixed spice
- Half cup of chopped dill
- Half cup of chopped cilantro
- Vegetable oil

Instructions:
1. Take a large bowl.
2. Add everything into the bowl and mix well.
3. Add water into the bowl to form a mixture.
4. Heat a frying pan and add vegetable oil in it.
5. Add a spoonful of batter to the pan carefully and cook them for few minutes.
6. Dish it out when fritters turn light brown in color.
7. Your dish is ready to be served.

6.10 Greek Chickpea Fritters Recipe

Preparation Time: 30 minutes
Cooking Time: 30 minutes
Serving: 4

Ingredients:

- One cup of parboiled chickpeas
- One cup of red onions
- One cup of gram flour
- A pinch of salt
- Two tablespoons of mixed spice
- Half cup of chopped dill
- Half cup of chopped cilantro
- Vegetable oil

Instructions:

1. Take a large bowl.
2. Add everything into the bowl and mix well.
3. Add water into the bowl to form a mixture.
4. Heat a frying pan and add vegetable oil in it.
5. Add a spoonful of batter to the pan carefully and cook them for few minutes.
6. Dish it out when fritters turn light brown in color.
7. Your dish is ready to be served.

6.11 Greek White Bean Stew Recipe

Preparation Time: 30 minutes
Cooking Time: 30 minutes
Serving: 4

Ingredients:

- One cup of chopped onions
- One cup of chopped parsley
- One cup of vegetable stock
- One cup of water
- A pinch of salt

- A pinch of black pepper
- Two tablespoons of olive oil
- One pound of white beans
- Half tablespoon of chopped garlic
- Two cups of chopped tomatoes
- Half cup of chopped fresh thyme
- Half cup of chopped fresh oregano
- Half cup of chopped fresh chives
- One teaspoon of mixed spice powder
- Half teaspoon of smoked paprika
- One bay leaf

Instructions:

1. Take a large pan.
2. Add the chopped onions and olive oil into it.
3. Mix the ingredients well.
4. Add the chopped garlic into the pan.
5. Add the tomatoes, oregano, bay leaf, salt, black pepper, thyme, smoked paprika, mix spice powder, and chives into the pan.
6. Cook the ingredients well.
7. Add the white beans into the mixture.
8. Add the vegetable stock and water into the pan.
9. Mix the stew well.
10. Place a lid on top of the pan.
11. Cook the stew for ten to fifteen minutes.
12. Dish out the stew when the beans are done.
13. Garnish the dish with chopped parsley on top.
14. Your dish is ready to be served.

6.12 Greek Vegetarian Bamies Recipe

Preparation Time: 30 minutes
Cooking Time: 30 minutes
Serving: 4

Ingredients:

- One cup of chopped onions
- One cup of chopped parsley

- One cup of vegetable stock
- One cup of water
- A pinch of salt
- A pinch of black pepper
- Two tablespoons of olive oil
- One pound of okra
- Half tablespoon of chopped garlic
- Two cups of chopped tomatoes
- Half cup of chopped fresh thyme
- Half cup of chopped fresh oregano
- Half cup of chopped fresh chives
- One teaspoon of mixed spice powder
- Half teaspoon of smoked paprika
- One bay leaf

Instructions:
1. Take a large pan.
2. Add the chopped onions and olive oil into it.
3. Mix the ingredients well.
4. Add the chopped garlic into the pan.
5. Add the tomatoes, oregano, bay leaf, salt, black pepper, thyme, smoked paprika, mix spice powder, and chives into the pan.
6. Cook the ingredients well.
7. Add the okra pieces into the mixture.
8. Add the vegetable stock and water into the pan.
9. Mix the stew well.
10. Place a lid on top of the pan.
11. Cook the stew for ten to fifteen minutes.
12. Dish out the stew when the vegetables are done.
13. Garnish the dish with chopped parsley on top.
14. Your dish is ready to be served.

6.13 Greek Grilled Vegetable Bowls Recipe

Preparation Time: 30 minutes
Cooking Time: 20 minutes
Serving: 4

Ingredients:

- One chopped red onion
- One cup of eggplant pieces
- One cup of zucchini pieces
- Two cups of cherry tomatoes
- Half cup of chopped parsley
- Two cups of feta cheese
- One cup of bell peppers
- One cup of mushrooms
- One cup of lemon dressing

Instructions:

1. Take a grill pan and add the olive oil in it.
2. Grill the vegetables on it.
3. Remove the vegetable when done.
4. Add the rest of the ingredients into the vegetables.
5. Mix everything well.
6. Your dish is ready to be served.

6.14 Greek Vegetable Balls with Tahini Lemon Sauce Recipe

Preparation Time: 10 minutes
Cooking Time: 20 minutes
Serving: 2

Ingredients:

- One chopped red onion
- Two minced garlic cloves
- A pinch of salt
- A pinch of black pepper
- Half cup of mint leaves
- Two cups of grated mixed vegetables
- Half teaspoon of oregano
- One egg
- Two tablespoons of olive oil
- One cup of tahini lemon sauce

Instructions:

1. Take a large bowl.
2. Add the grated mixed vegetables, spices, mint, onion, garlic, and egg into the bowl.
3. Mix all the ingredients well and form round ball structures.
4. Fry the vegetable balls in olive oil until they turn golden brown.
5. Dish out the balls.
6. Serve the balls with tahini lemon sauce on the side.
7. Your dish is ready to be served.

Preparation Time: 30 minutes
Cooking Time: 30 minutes
Serving: 4

Ingredients:

- Half cup of chopped parsley
- Two tablespoons of oregano leaves
- One tablespoon of rosemary leaves
- Two tablespoons of parsley leaves
- Half cup of chopped onion
- Two tablespoons of olive oil
- Half cup of basil leaves
- One tablespoon of crushed red pepper
- Half teaspoon of fennel leaves
- A pinch of kosher salt
- A pinch of black pepper
- Three cups of mixed vegetable pieces
- One cup of chopped chives
- One cup of cherry tomatoes
- Half cup of savory summer sprigs
- Two tablespoons of minced garlic
- Two tablespoons of dried thyme

Instructions:

1. Take a large pan.
2. Add the olive oil and chopped onions into it.
3. Cook the onions until they turn light brown in color.
4. Add the minced garlic into the pan.
5. Cook the mixture for five minutes.
6. Season the mixture with salt and pepper.
7. Add the spices and all the vegetables.
8. In a bowl, crush the cherry tomatoes and add the salt.
9. Dish the mixture out in a plate when the vegetables are done.
10. Add the crushed tomatoes into the pan.
11. Cook the tomatoes for ten minutes or until they turn soft.
12. Add the vegetable mixture into the pan again.
13. Add the rest of the ingredients into the pan and bake it for about fifteen minutes.

14. Your dish is ready to be served.

6.16 Greek Aborigine and Tomato Stew Recipe

Preparation Time: 30 minutes
Cooking Time: 30 minutes
Serving: 4

Ingredients:

- One cup of chopped onions
- One cup of chopped parsley
- One cup of vegetable stock
- One cup of water
- A pinch of salt
- A pinch of black pepper
- Two tablespoons of olive oil
- One pound of aborigine
- Half tablespoon of chopped garlic
- Two cups of chopped tomatoes
- Half cup of chopped fresh thyme
- Half cup of chopped fresh oregano
- Half cup of chopped fresh chives
- One teaspoon of mixed spice powder
- Half teaspoon of smoked paprika
- One bay leaf

Instructions:

1. Take a large pan.
2. Add the chopped onions and olive oil into it.
3. Mix the ingredients well.
4. Add the chopped garlic into the pan.
5. Add the tomatoes, oregano, bay leaf, salt, black pepper, thyme, smoked paprika, mix spice powder, and chives into the pan.
6. Cook the ingredients well.
7. Add the aborigine into the mixture.
8. Add the vegetable stock and water into the pan.
9. Mix the stew well.
10. Place a lid on top of the pan.
11. Cook the stew for ten to fifteen minutes.

12. Dish out the stew when the vegetables are done.
13. Garnish the dish with chopped parsley on top.
14. Your dish is ready to be served.

6.17 Greek Avocado Tartine Recipe

Preparation Time: 30 minutes
Cooking Time: 20 minutes
Serving: 4

Ingredients:

- Half cup of lemon juice
- Four slices of Tartine bread
- Half cup of cherry tomatoes
- Half cup of extra-virgin olive oil
- Half cup of crumbled cheese
- Crushed red chilies
- A quarter cup of dill
- Two cups of chopped avocado
- A pinch of salt
- A pinch of black pepper

Instructions:
1. Take a large bowl.
2. Add all the ingredients except the bread slices.
3. Mix all the ingredients.
4. Toast the tartine bread slices
5. Spread the mixture on top of the bread slices.
6. Your dish is ready to be served.

6.18 Greek Spinach Rice Recipe

Preparation Time: 10 minutes
Cooking Time: 20 minutes
Serving: 2

Ingredients:

- Three cups of chopped spinach

- Two teaspoons of lemon juice
- Half cup of chopped onions
- Two tablespoons of minced garlic
- Two tablespoons of olive oil
- A pinch of salt
- A pinch of black pepper
- A quarter cup of dried mint
- Two tablespoons of chopped fresh dill
- Two pounds of rice grains
- Two cups of tomato paste
- Two cups of water

Instructions:
1. Take a large saucepan.
2. Add the water into the pan and season it with salt.
3. Boil the water and then add the rice into the water.
4. Boil the rice and then drain it.
5. Take a large pan.
6. Add the olive oil and heat it well.
7. Add the chopped onions into the pan and cook it until it turns soft and fragrant.
8. Add the chopped garlic into the pan.
9. Add the spinach, tomato paste, lemon juice, salt, and crushed black pepper into the pan.
10. Cook the ingredients for about ten minutes.
11. Add the boiled rice into the pan and mix well.
12. Add the dried mint and chopped dill into the pan.
13. Place a lid on top of the pan.
14. Cook the rice for about five minutes on low heat.
15. Your dish is ready to be served.

6.19 Greek Avgolemono Soup Recipe

Preparation Time: 30 minutes
Cooking Time: 30 minutes
Serving: 4

Ingredients:

- Half cup of chopped fresh thyme

- Half cup of chopped fresh oregano
- Half cup of chopped fresh chives
- One teaspoon of mixed spice powder
- Half teaspoon of smoked paprika
- One bay leaf
- A pinch of salt
- A pinch of black pepper
- Two tablespoons of olive oil
- One pound of chicken pieces
- Half tablespoon of chopped garlic
- Two cups of chopped tomatoes
- One cup of chopped onions
- One cup of chopped parsley
- One cup of vegetable stock
- One cup of water
- Half cup of lemon juice

Instructions:

1. Take a large pan.
2. Add the chopped onions and olive oil into it.
3. Mix the ingredients well.
4. Add the chopped garlic into the pan.
5. Add the tomatoes, oregano, bay leaf, salt, black pepper, thyme, smoked paprika, mix spice powder, and chives into the pan.
6. Cook the ingredients well.
7. Add the chicken pieces and lemon juice into the mixture.
8. Add the vegetable stock and water into the pan.
9. Mix the soup well.
10. Place a lid on top of the pan.
11. Cook the soup for ten to fifteen minutes.
12. Dish out the soup when the chicken pieces are done.
13. Garnish the dish with chopped parsley on top.
14. Your dish is ready to be served.

6.20 Greek Vegetable Pitas Recipe

Preparation Time: 10 minutes
Cooking Time: 15 minutes
Serving: 2

Ingredients:

- Two tablespoons of olive oil
- Two pieces of pita breads
- Two large eggs
- One ripe cherry tomato
- Two cups of mixed vegetables
- One cup of chopped onion
- Half cup of chopped basil
- A quarter cup of crumbled feta cheese
- A pinch of salt
- A pinch of black pepper
- A bunch of chopped cilantro

Instructions:

1. Take a large pan.
2. Add the olive oil into the pan.
3. Add the onion and salt into the pan.
4. Cook the onions well and then add the black pepper into the pan.
5. Add the mixed vegetables into the mixture.
6. Add the chopped basil into the mixture.
7. Cook the ingredients well for about fifteen minutes.
8. Dish out when the vegetables are done.
9. Let the meat cool down, and then add the crumbled feta cheese into it.
10. Mix well.
11. Heat the pita bread.
12. Cut a hole into the bread and add the cooked mixture into it.
13. Garnish the bread with chopped cilantro.
14. Your dish is ready to be served.

Conclusion

The establishment of Greek cooking lies in the dietary patterns of Southern European nations, explicitly the Mediterranean nations. Mediterranean gastronomy is based to a great extent around natural products, entire grains, and lean protein like fish and chicken. In Greece, proteins from non-meat sources like beans and vegetables are additionally well known in soups, stews, and mixed greens.

This book covers the life of a Greek, making it easy for them to prepare their favourite recipes inside their kitchen without any stress. This cookbook incorporates 75 healthy plans that contain breakfast recipes, lunch and dinner recipes, snack recipes, dessert recipes, and vegetarian recipes that you can undoubtedly make at home very easily. So, start cooking today with this amazing and easy cookbook.

www.ingramcontent.com/pod-product-compliance
Lightning Source LLC
Chambersburg PA
CBHW080627030426
42336CB00018B/3112